I0413197

HER

Inner Games

of Sex

(An Appraisal of Female Sex Problems – with Solutions)

By

Dr Harry Howell

This book has been transcribed directly from one of my seminars for health care practitioners in order to try and capture the spirit of audience participation, rather than write it in the usual stodgy fashion.

I usually begin by strolling up and down at the front of the hall delivering my concepts, from which the students will get ample opportunity to ask any questions which will allow us to expand on the subject.

The Royal Masonic Hospital, London

You don't have to have seen 'When Harry Met Sally' to know what an orgasm is. That particular clip has been shown so many times that everyone knows what I mean. But what does it all really mean?

That young lady, standing on the street corner, with her legs crossed, shivering and shuddering away could mean a lot of things. She could be cold. She might need to spend a penny. Or she might have seen a guy so stunning that she had an instant orgasm.

But more than that, it raises the question, If it's so easy for a woman to have an orgasm, does it mean that every female we see who has her legs crossed and is squirming just a little bit, is on the point of an orgasmic explosion? Wow! What a thought. I mean, they're everywhere, these orgasming women. Until Sally came along, we never knew what it meant. Now we're surrounded by orgasms.

So while we've got this burgeoning development among the females, the poor old men – well, not necessarily old – are going through the opposite situation. While men used to be able to orgasm at the sight of a pretty pair of legs, now they are finding it more and more difficult to achieve the same thing after an hour's foreplay. Even the 'wet dream' has become a 'wet nightmare', because they hardly ever happen any more.

Something's going wrong somewhere.

Women don't wank ... they 'pleasure themselves'. Wanking is only for men. In Victorian England, the age of the 'double standards', women were regarded as little more than playthings for men, not entitled to any sexual pleasures of their own, and certainly not capable of homosexuality. A little more than a hundred years later and we see women quickly becoming the dominant sexual force.

Go into any Ann Summers shop and most of the stuff displayed around you is for females. Things to wear – ranging from delicate black lingerie to black leather gear and whips – and an enormous panoply of sex toys for women. Far from denying that they ever masturbated – as they did a few decades ago – they are proud to tell all and sundry of their latest sexploits, which frequently don't include men.

Vibrators are undoubtedly the biggest selling sex toy, and they come in an immense range of products and styles. Some have at least seven different speeds, they vibrate at different levels, they can pulse, they can have attachments that enable them to reach the G-spot, they can be skin-safe and waterproof, some have 'ears' (like the '*Rabbit*') that tickle or pulse the clitoris while they thrust and penetrate deep inside … in fact it is almost impossible to think of anything that could be done that hasn't been done to ensure complete satisfaction for a female.

The first mechanical vibrator was invented in 1869 by an American physician, and this was prescribed for women with hysteria, anxieties, and excessive wetness. It's an often overlooked fact than in Victorian times physicians were quite frequently inclined to masturbate a female to orgasm to prove her capacity to achieve one. These actions, including the mechanical vibrator – which often broke down at a critical moment, rather like the battery running flat at the moment of climax – were deemed necessary because it was regarded as unfitting for women of esteem to masturbate themselves. If ever a man became dispensable, it might be said the development and popularity of the vibrator has brought about his downfall.

Dildos have long been used by women. For centuries, reindeers' horns were used by women in Scandinavia. The earliest dildo on record dates back to the Upper Palaeolithic age – that's 30,000 years ago – when a siltstone phallus was found in some caves near Ulm in Germany that could hardly have been used for any other purpose. Archaeologists have unearthed many a dildo from excavations in Egypt, and Greek vases have depicted the use of dildos several hundred years BC.

Greek literature was also splattered with frank references to the use of dildos, and comic plays by Herodas and Aristophanes spoke freely of their leather dildos in language that would be too flagrant to use two-and-a-half thousand years after they were written. The ancient Chinese used wooden dildos, though earlier dildos had been made from stone and even tar. Africans frequently used dildos made from camel dung and coated with a resin. The need for penetration had obviously been recognised thousands of years ago, although this wasn't only used for masturbation and was often employed in deflowering virgins either as sacrifice to gods or in preparation for marriage.

Chastity before marriage hasn't always been recognised as a virtue. Interestingly, a 2000 year-old brothel was excavated recently in Athens, and within the brothel was a 'sex shop' area which still had stock in it, including vaginal and anal dildos and various other sex toys. In Zanzibar, two hundred years ago, a wooden dildo with double ends was found, showing that the use of a single dildo by two female partners had been established even that long ago. In this country, it is difficult to trace the history of dildos, but Ben Johnson wrote about them in *The Alchemist* in 1610, and a year later William Shakespeare made mention of them in *The Winter's Tale* (Act 4, Scene iv, line 196): 'so without bawdry, which is strange; with such delicate burthens of dildos and fadings, "jump her and thump her"'.

The modern dildo has undergone some modifications in terms of materials, size and shape. Also, there are strap-on dildos, which enable lesbians to play the role of the male and indulge in female-to-female intercourse. I have had more than one male patient who has worn a strap-on dildo with his wife because his own penis was too small to give any satisfaction, or simply because he was unable to achieve or maintain an erection for long enough. Some females use a strap-on dildo to penetrate a male anus, a practise called 'pegging'. Some sex shops have rooms or cubicles where a female can be hitched up to a – I almost hesitate to use the term, but it *is* the actual name of the product – Fucking Machine. This is a contraption with a piston-type rod that has a phallus-shaped rubber penis on the end. It can be fitted into the vagina or anus (in some cases *both simultaneously*) and it thrusts in and out at varying speeds that can be controlled by the user. It is almost the ultimate sex toy, except it is too expensive for home use.

I say *almost* the ultimate, because there are other methods either in use now or in varying stages of development. For example, there is a new product called the ShockSpot Fucking System that controls stroke length, speed and smoothness of action at the touch of a button on your PC, laptop or palm button. You can even store and share your programmes with other users on the internet. It fits into a case not much larger than a briefcase and will accommodate almost any position, including lying, kneeling, seating or standing. It is portable, obviously, and can be taken to parties where all your friends can try it out for everybody's fun. What a changing world!

There is a product called *Sinulator*, in which you hook up your sex toy to the internet, which enables other people around the world to control its actions. For example, you can link-up your vibrator or dildo to the internet and have someone in Hong Kong or Brasilia or Cape Town control its speed, depth of penetration, vibration-rate etc., and also decide if you are to orgasm quickly, drawn-out, stop at the critical moment or not orgasm at all. This is called *Cybersex* and is becoming increasingly popular.

Other sex toys include the so-called *Chinese Eggs*, which consist of a couple of oval-shaped balls which are inserted into the vagina where they vibrate according to body movements, thus stimulating throughout the day. There is one called the Radio Love Vibrating Egg which is radio-controlled so that you vary the speed and rate of vibration via a remote control. You can, if you wish, hand the remote control to a partner and entrust them to regulate your 'egg' through to orgasm.

So, the message is, female sex has widened out from those dark Victorian days so that just about anything goes today. And females have moved from not daring to even whisper about their sexual mores to openly discussing it, even to promoting it on the internet through an abundance of websites and social networks specialising in this. And with the development of mobile phones that incorporate photo and video facilities, it is not uncommon for females and males to take quick photos of themselves in various poses and stages of undress and nakedness and upload them straight on the internet so that others can see them.

Something that caught my eye recently was the concept of chastity belts. These were said to have been originally developed for the Crusading Knights, so that they wouldn't have to worry about other men taking advantage of their loved ones while they were away fighting a war on our behalf that practically no one else wanted – rather like today, I sense. But what's new is that we now have chastity belts for men! And a surprising number of females are employing them on their partner. To me they look as gruesome as the old female cast iron belts, although the male counterparts are usually plastic or made of cord. But is their need real or imagined?

Watersports has become a developing theme. For some there has always been a curiosity of how the other gender passes water. It was never that uncommon for a female to get a kick out of holding a penis while the partner urinates, nor did males conceal their desire to watch a female passing water. But the advent of the internet has thrown all these things wide open to anybody who wants to log in. What is relatively new is the game of urinating over a partner, male or female. Or even groups of people urinating over a sacrificial-like victim.

This has led on to another growing phenomenon –

squirting. That is, on the right stimulation, a female releasing what some see as an ejaculation and others see as a form of urinating during sex play or intercourse. Certainly it varies between females from a drip to a gentle stream or even a raging squirt that can reach several feet across a room. So what is it? An ejaculation or merely urine? Well, it is neither. Certainly it is not urine, too many clinical tests have been carried out to refute that. Nor is it strictly speaking an ejaculation – at least in the sense of being comparable to a male ejaculation.

Stag nights for men go back a long way, centuries, in fact. But the equivalent for females, the 'hens' night, only dates back to the 1960s. And since then has seen a series of changes. What started as a girls' night out as they gave their bride-to-be friend a final fling before the marriage usually scheduled for the following day, in which quantities of booze would be consumed while watching and cheering a male stripper to the sound of raucous music, has become a bawdy night of sexual revelries that could include literal orgies taking place – sometimes including the bride-to-be.

This has led to a complete new industry springing up, usually within the all-embracing sobriquet of cfnm (clothed female/s naked male/s). Hordes of websites have sprung up like handkerchiefs at a bullfight just dealing with this one theme. Clubs and organisations have also arisen, one of the chief ones being *Dancing Bear*, in which large groups of women sit and drink booze while men appear, partially clad, to the sound of loud, vibrant music. To the cheers of women in varying stages of intoxication urging the man or men to 'get 'em off' – a phrase previously thought belonged only to men – as the male/s begin to do just that. They would then pass along the rows of women, stopping off to allow themselves to be fondled, even fellated, and sometimes – especially as the evening wore on – to be enticed into actual sexual intercourse. All this performed to the vociferous encouragement of the female audience. Of course, there's nothing really new about all this – it was quite common in the days of Emperor Nero, although he himself would probably have been in another saloon being entertained by young boys not yet into their teens.

Another development has been in the area of male ejaculations and the female. It has often been the case – reputed to have come about because of the Roman Catholic Church's opposition to condoms – that a male has withdrawn just prior to orgasm and allowed his semen to be directed to various parts of the female anatomy. This could be aimed at the buttocks, the genital area, the stomach, the breasts or even the face, including the mouth. The face seems to have become an ever-favoured place, giving rise to the term 'facials'. Then the new game of bukakke developed, in which different men lined up in turn to ejaculate over a female's face – with the female in question urging them to give her more and more, as though a gallon or two were insufficient. A far distant cry from those not-too-long-ago days when sex often took place between two people in a darkened room – with scarcely a sound uttered until, perhaps, that very last moment of climax.

You might be wondering what all this has to do with female problems. I seem to have talked about nothing but female behaviour and how it has developed over the last decades or so. Well, there are problems attached to all these behaviours, as I hope will come out when we get to the questions time. But in case any of you have been thinking along these lines, some of the age-old questions still remain – often unanswered, unfortunately.

I have mentioned frigidity, which is one. There is also painful intercourse, which can arise from different reasons – some of them physical, some of them psychological. Menstrual difficulties, including menopause, affect millions of females and may often have a simple solution. Infertility is yet another problem for a large number of females, and interestingly this number is growing – statistically – which might have sinister undertones to it.

Homosexuality, lesbianism, has become much less of a problem as society has become more open to it, but problems do still remain for many females in this area, particularly as some may feel that they were born the 'wrong' sex. So gender identity is a real problem for some females, as it is indeed for many males who feel they are legally male but should be female. Some problems are of a legal nature, others of a cultural nature, and yet others might be nothing more than psychological – which can be real enough for those concerned.

So, let's see where all this leads us as we throw the whole subject open to your questions.

ON A MORE SERIOUS NOTE

CYBIL: I'm somewhat surprised in your opening address that you didn't even mention really serious problems like cancer of the breasts, or cancer of the ovaries. I'm sorry if we have to cross swords over this but these problems are so much more serious than whether a female masturbates or not.

HH: I understand what you're saying, Cybil, and we won't have to cross swords at all. The reason I haven't mentioned the various types of cancers is because they don't come under this theme of female sexual problems. They come under the theme of Disease. I could, of course, have mentioned Aids and other sexually transmitted diseases which are the direct result of sexual activity but I try to leave some things unsaid so that they can come spontaneously from the audience. [Cybil shrugs and nods]

FRANCES: I also want to mention something that you

didn't talk about. Women's breasts. I don't mean illnesses like cancer but the question of shape and size. Isn't it true to say that so many women don't actually like their breasts and a whole new industry has grown up to cater for them?

HH: Yes, a very valid point. It's all very nice females having fantastic breasts while they're young, but when they start having children their breasts often begin to change shape and all kinds of things can go wrong with them. Droopiness is one thing. Becoming over-large is another. And I'm sure we are all aware of things that can – but not necessarily do – go wrong with breast implants, and so on. But I don't think you actually asked me a question, Frances. So where do you want this to go?

FRANCES: I don't know. It's just that you hadn't mentioned breasts, yet they are one of the biggest problems facing a whole lot of women. Would you recommend breast enhancement of any kind?

HH: I wouldn't, actually. I think that it's more of a

psychological problem than physical. I know that there are many, many females who would like larger breasts. Yet somehow, I get the feeling that it isn't because they really do want larger breasts but because they want to satisfy a partner who wants them to have bigger breasts ... or maybe because they feel that, if they don't have a partner, maybe it's because their breasts are too small. The reality is, there are many men out there who actually prefer smaller breasts. And the same applies to lesbians: not all lesbians want large breasts on their partner. So for those females who think small breasts are holding back their love life, let me assure them it just isn't so. There might be other reasons they haven't found a partner. Women who do have larger breasts don't necessarily have men flocking around them.

So the message really is this: we should each learn to, at the very least, *accept* the body we have. We could, if we wanted, learn to love what we've got. I always think of Shakespeare's words in this connection: 'Nothing is good or bad but thinking makes it so.' And that sums it up perfectly. It's not the size of the breasts but the way we think about them. And that applies to any other part of the body.

I have a specific questionnaire for sexual problems and one of the questions … in fact, it's not just one question, it's a series of questions in which I ask them along these lines: 'What do you think of your hair?' What do you think of your eyes? The colour, shape, etc.' And I work my way down the body, including the breasts, the genitals, the knees, legs, feet, and so on. Frances has pointed out dissatisfaction with breasts, but other women – and men, too – might be dissatisfied with another part of their body. The nose is a common one. Once you know a person is unhappy about a particular body part, you can then work on it. Whether people have chided them on it, made nasty comments, and so on.

It isn't difficult to find examples of other people

who haven't suffered, even though they might have had a similar problem. Women with small breasts … I could say, 'Well, Audrey Hepburn had small breasts. So do Kate Hudson, Juliette Binoche and Keira Knightly. Nicole Kidman also has small breasts. And none of them have done badly. They've carved out great screen careers and, as far as I know, have had lots of men yearning for them. So, small breasts don't have to be a problem.'

Having a large nose doesn't have to be a problem, either. It never stood in Barry Manilow's way. Dustin Hoffman and Tony Bennett don't seem to have suffered. Barbra Streisand, Sarah Jessica Parker, Bette Midler, Jennifer Aniston are all said to have a large nose, yet they've all done well in life. It isn't difficult, when you think about it, to give a good logical reason why no kind of handicap has to be a handicap. And if logic doesn't work, you can always suggest hypnotherapy, which is an excellent way of making a person come to terms with their body.

FRANCES: That was a much better answer than I was hoping for. Thank you, Harry. [loud applause]

HH: I might just add that I think there are some *special* cases where surgery can be of help. I'm thinking perhaps of some people who actually do need breast reduction, but these are exceptions and not for every woman who feels her breasts are too big. As for breast enlargement, I've never really met a needy case. I don't like the idea of a woman carrying a bag of synthetic gel in her chest cavity. I know that materials have improved, surgery has improved, but I think natural is nearly always best. Most of the cases that I've seen of breast enhancement … they look so unnatural. I confess I have never been in the position of handling an enhanced breast but I imagine it would be like feeling a foam rubber pillow.

SYLVIA: Can we get away from frivolous questions and get on …

HH: Hold on, Sylvia. Why are you calling them

frivolous? These are serious concern to a lot of females.

SYLVIA: I wasn't referring to the question on breasts, more about sex toys and that sort of thing.

HH: Sex toys have become part of life and they actually perform a useful function for a lot of people. They open up areas of sexuality that had been closed to them hitherto.

SYLVIA: Well, there are different ways of looking at things.

HH: So which way do you look at things?

SYLVIA: I like to see sex from a moral point of view. As a practising Christian, and I know I am probably in a minority here, but I still think that the purpose of sex is to procreate children. It's not about inventing games to play just to make sex good fun. Having sex for the right reason does give fun, and a great inner satisfaction, in itself.

HH: Okay, and I think we all respect your view on that, but in the same way you should also respect the right of others to have their views, even though they are different from your own.

SYLVIA:　But that is what is taking society down a slippery slope to ruin. We have seen throughout history how empires have fallen into degeneracy and decay. What happened in Rome is happening here in the so-called civilised world. Pornography and corruption are destroying our society and we are all standing by and letting it happen.

HH:　Okay, you've made your point, whether we all agree with it or not. Do you have a question related to female sexual problems or have you said what you wanted?

SYLVIA:　I do have a question. It relates to frigidity.

HH:　Alfred Kinsey once said, 'There are no frigid women, only inept men.' Do you have a specific question?

SYLVIA:　Yes. What treatments are there for frigidity?

HH:　Most of the causes of frigidity within women are psychogenic. It is a condition in which women are generally

25

unresponsive to sexual stimulation, and who generally attain little or no erotic pleasure. It is not to be confused with sexual anaesthesia, in which a female may actually enjoy sexual contact with a male although unable to actually enjoy a sensation of touch. In physiological terms, the normal female response to stimulation would be vaginal lubrication, swelling and colouration of the vaginal walls, engorgement of the clitoris, and formation of the orgasmic platform.

With *General Sexual Dysfunction* – a long-winded term generally preferred to frigidity – these physical responses are lacking, although it is possible for an orgasm to be experienced despite these impairments.

- *Primary* frigidity refers to a female who has never had intercourse, and has never experienced erotic pleasure with any partner at any time.

- *Secondary* frigidity refers to one who has had intercourse or erotic pleasure at some time.

- *Tertiary* frigidity applies to a female who is sexually unresponsive to her husband or normal partner but can enjoy sex with another partner.

In Primary cases, there is often a case of repressive upbringing, either by strict parents or for orthodox religious reasons. Occasionally, it is as the result of a frightening childhood experience, e.g. child molesting, witnessing something unpleasant (mother having sex with stranger, exposure of penis, perhaps in a threatening way, by a stranger), or even a male sibling, uncle or father who has behaved in some sexual manner towards her. It may also be the result of a hysteric personality disorder.

Secondary cases, much more common and diverse in causative factors, can often be traced back to a child-birth, not necessarily the first, tiredness or depression, living in crowded conditions, may be concerned about becoming pregnant, menstrual irregularity or pain – *dysmennorhoea* – or feelings of resentment towards husband or partner, to name just a few.

Factors which reduce erotic interest for a female include:

- lack of sexual interest in partner

- inadequate stimulation

- poor communication with partner

- anxiety or acute tension

- shame/guilt due to restrictive upbringing or religious beliefs

- fear of losing control

- fear of rejection through failure to satisfy partner

- fear of pregnancy

- fear of partner (perhaps aggressive, sadistic, brutal, heavy drinker, etc.)

- will permit sex only out of marital duty

As a result of any of these characteristics, the female protects herself by erecting a defensive barrier. The job of therapy is to penetrate the barrier and reach the areas of sensitivity beneath.

Sexual attraction, the ability to have orgasms, and many other sexual characteristics, are essentially a question of culture. Sudanese, Ethiopian, and many other African countries have a custom of female circumcision – usually illegal but nevertheless still practised – which is a device to prevent a woman from having an orgasm. The recognised role of such women is to bear children.

In our own culture, within the last few years, sex has been discussed more openly than at any time within the last century. Improved methods of contraception have meant that many more women are now predisposed to have sex for its own sake, and they feel – quite rightly – that they are entitled to be able to enjoy it.

But there are still many other factors that can

prevent a female from enjoying sex. She may be physically attracted to a partner but regard him as stupid, coarse, or unintelligent. She may wish to reward him on some occasions and punish him on others. Sex, in fact, is often used as a bargaining factor within a relationship – even a marital one.

There is also the question of leading and dominance. Some females prefer to be led, others to lead. She may have contempt for a partner lacking expertise, or who is selfish sexually. Or she may wish to totally dominate a man or, conversely, be totally dominated. If a partner is contrary to any of these deeply felt desires, the result may be a total disinterest in sex or a particular partner. Some women prefer 'gentle' lovers, others prefer their partner to be more forceful, or manly. Some prefer younger men, others the older type.

Some women even set out to be 'vengeful' on *all* men in return for some historical event causing them unhappiness. The role of the father may be important here, if one is looking for historical causes. Some women are able to appear passionate and willing simply in order to enable their partner to ejaculate quickly – even before penetration, perhaps – and thus bring a quick end to the ordeal.

Unlike men, who are rarely affected sexually through hormone imbalance, this is somewhat more likely with females, and there are a number of cases where an increase in *testosterone* has a definite effect.

The principal female sex hormones are androgen and oestrogen, and it has been discovered that females seem to lose all sexual interest when the source of androgen production is removed by surgery. When given testosterone, however, they become highly sexually aroused. Because it is essentially a male sex hormone, and only produced in females in small quantities, care has to be taken to avoid masculinising side-effects, e.g. hirsutism (excess body or facial hair).

Physical, medical and organic causes for lowering sexual desire within females includes the following:

- infections

- any chronic painful illness

- renal, pulmonary and cardiac diseases

- malignancies

- advanced stages of diabetes

- dyspareunia

- vaginismus

- ovarian tumours and cysts

- anal fissures

- haemorrhoids

- vaginal polyps

- prolapsed uterus

- any inflammation of the pelvis

With post-partum secondary frigidity, a good clue is the post-natal examination, usually about 6 weeks after birth. If a female indicates to her partner that she wants to wait until after the examination before renewing intercourse it is often the case that general sexual dysfunction is taking place.

I just want to mention a couple of related questions that arise.

Hypoactive sexual desire disorder is regarded as the most common sexual problem for women. Criteria necessary for this diagnosis include persistently deficient or absent sexual fantasies and/or desire for sexual activity.

This must be considered in cases where the lack of sexual interest causes marked distress or interpersonal difficulty. The first enquiry here must be to eliminate any organic problems as a possible cause. The most likely cause is a hormone deficiency, especially testosterone, or DHEA – *dehydroepiandrosterone*. The next one to test for is

33

serotonin.

Sexual aversion disorder is where a female avoids any sexual contact, usually of a genital nature, although in rare cases this can include kissing or even touching.

The effect, when confronted with a sexual opportunity is usually anxiety, fear or disgust. This condition generally affects females who have been through some type of sexual crisis, such as rape, gang rape, forced sex, or sex with a family member. This disorder is also very common in some religions as some faiths have very strict rules about sexual activity.

Lack of lubrication can also be a cause of female frigidity. This is a condition often seen in young women, and in those cases is nearly always caused as a side effect of birth control pills or shots.

Another cause can be diabetes, especially in long-standing cases. This would also cause lack of blood to the sex organs, which could result in fungal or bacterial infections of the nether regions.

Radiation treatments can also cause lack of lubrication. This may be due to treatment for breast lumps or cancer. The drug Tamoxifen can also cause dryness. Vitamin E suppositories can be helpful in these cases.

Dryness of the vagina is also seen in breast-feeding mothers, due to a high elevation of prolactin, which can also cause a lack of interest in sex.

So, eliminating all these variables is important. Testing and treating the Bartholin glands, which we'll talk about when we come to Dyspareunia, as I'm sure we will, is one approach. When everything fails, synthetic lubrication can be considered. Only water-soluble lubricants should be used as they don't usually create new problems. Silicon lubricants are also usually problem-free. But avoid all petroleum-based lubricants, such as Vaseline. They're sticky, and can harbour bacteria.

FRANK: You mentioned a questionnaire. Do you have one for frigidity?

HH: Yes, and I'm going to hand them round right now. [Questionnaires handed round. For the benefit of readers, below is printed the identical questionnaire]

QUESTIONNAIRE

Sexual Attitudes

1. Do you believe you have a basic human right to enjoy sex?

2. Is the main purpose of sex to produce children, or for pleasure?

3. Do you find some sexual practices disgusting?

4. Are you willing to try anything at least once?

5. Do you believe that a male should dominate sexually?

6. Do you believe it is a woman's duty to please her

partner sexually?

7.   Do you feel sexually attracted towards your partner?

8.   Do you hold any religious convictions regarding sex?

Outline of Dysfunctions

1.   Under what circumstances have you experienced an orgasm, if ever?

2.   Has your sexual relationship with present partner been happy? If not, at what point did it become unsatisfactory?

3.   How long have you had this relationship?

4.   What previous relationships have you had?

5.   Did you experience sexual satisfaction or not?

6.   Has your partner tried means other than intercourse to bring sexual pleasure to you? Describe.

7.   Describe your first sexual experience within the present relationship.

8. Are the non-sexual areas of your relationship satisfactory? Describe.

9. Have you participated in any extra-marital activities within this relationship? If so, have they been sexually satisfying?

10. If so, is your partner aware of them?

11. To your knowledge, has your partner indulged in any extra-marital activities?

12. Has your partner experienced any erectile or ejaculatory difficulty?

13. Have you, at any time, experienced sexual happiness? Describe.

Sexual Development

1. At what age did you first experience a genital feeling of pleasure?

2. At what age did you first experiment with masturbation?

3. How did you first learn about masturbation?

4. How frequently did you pursue masturbation?

5. Have you masturbated during the present relationship (a) with partner's knowledge? (b) without partner's knowledge?

6. Do you experience orgasm (a) through masturbation (b) through intercourse (c) not at all?

7. Do you enjoy being touched by partner?

8. If no to previous question, was there ever a time when you did enjoy being touched by partner?

9. What prevents your enjoyment of it now?

10. What was your principal attraction to your partner?

11. Is that attraction still there today?

12. Have you ever been asked to perform a sexual act you regard as disgusting?

13. Have you ever been forced to perform a sexual act you find disgusting?

14. How frequently did you have intercourse in the early part of this present relationship?

15. Was that frequency satisfactory to you?

16. What frequency might you have preferred, given the choice?

Medical

1. Have you ever had any surgery? Describe.

2. Have you ever had any serious illness? Which?

3. Have you ever been treated for depression? If so, what treatment was prescribed? Note any of the following medications: methadone, morphine, ravell, codeine, heroine (all have a depressive action on the Central Nervous System)

Sexual Behaviour

1. Does lovemaking usually lead to intercourse?

2. Where does sex usually take place?

3. At what time of day?

4. Who has the greatest influence on sex, you or your partner?

5. What turns you on most?

6. What turns you off most?

7. Are you able to discuss sex openly with partner?

8. Does your partner have any sexual habits you dislike?

9. Does your partner stimulate you adequately?

10. Do you ever fear losing control of yourself during sex?

11. Are you concerned about failing to satisfy your partner?

12. Do you ever worry about becoming pregnant? Frequently?

13. Does your partner frighten you sometimes?

14. How do you feel about touching partner's genitals?

15. How do you feel about partner touching your genitals?

16. Do you place any limitations on partner (i.e. Not to touch certain parts)?

17. Do you ever fake an orgasm to please partner? Frequently?

Body Image

1. What do you think of your hair? Style, texture, colour?

2. How about your eyes?

3. Nose. Are you satisfied with it?

4. Would you like it changed in any way?

5. How about your mouth? Are you satisfied with it?

6. Voice. How do you feel about your voice?

7. What about your arms?

8. How about your hands?

9. Your overall figure. What do you think about it? Height, weight, etc.

10. How about your breasts? Are they too big, too small, too saggy?

11. And the nipples. How do you feel about them?

12. Are your breasts and nipples sensitive to touch?

13. How about your stomach? How do you feel about your stomach?

14. And how about your hips?

15. Genitals. How do you feel about your genitals?

16. How about your pubic hair? Are you conscious of it?

17. Do you feel that your vagina is too small? Too tight? Too loose?

18. How about your clitoris? Is it sensitive to touch?

19. Do you try to avoid exposing your genitals to anyone? To partner?

20. What about your buttocks? Satisfied?

21. Thighs. How do you feel about your thighs?

22. Legs?

23. Feet? Satisfied with your feet? And your toes?

24. How about your personality? How do you feel about that?

25. How do you feel about your partner's body?

Ideal

1. Can you describe how you think a sexual encounter should be?

2. Have you ever experienced anything like that?

3. Do you think it is possible to achieve the ideal?

4. What things are you good at (sexually)?

5. What things are you not good at (sexually)?

It's really important to recognise that we, as therapists, do not sit in judgement. There are no right or wrong answers to any of the above questions. They are only asked in order to provide enough information to enable us to determine how to proceed … which are the areas that need to be developed to give us a clearer understanding where the source of a problem might lie.

Because women often use sex as a weapon – they frequently find it's the only weapon they have – there is sometimes a tendency to look negatively at the whole purpose of sex. They are threatened and coerced sexually during their childhood, and underlying sexual tensions lead them to associate sex with fear. This, together with the fact that sex has virtually been controlled by men, means that females often feel that they are little more than 'sexual objects' in the eyes of men, to be exploited and used, and very often just dumped when that usefulness is over.

It is often considered all right for men to have a little sex on the side, a night out at a strip show, a stag night, and so on. Society is changing in its attitudes towards sex but only slowly, and for some women not at all. So male therapists, in particular, need to understand and accept that sex in the minds of many, if not most, females is not the same as in the eyes of men. While boys in adolescence often get some encouragement from father to go out and get some experience, many adolescent girls get strict warnings from mother. This might be particularly severe in cases where mother herself has been sexually suppressed and victimised.

These childhood warnings can become deeply imprinted and prevent normal sexual release. Masturbation might have been regarded as something dirty, and even the naked body itself to be scarcely looked at, even by its owner. So one often finds, in therapy, that there is a reluctance to talk about body images, masturbation, and other similar topics of a very personal nature.

Inhibitions of feeling can often be quickly detected by inhibitions of breathing, so we can use deep breathing to help people get down to deep feelings. And increased awareness of body is important. Client should be urged to start taking more note of her body, perhaps standing in front of a full-length mirror and carefully observing every part of herself, gently touching each part to see how much sensitivity exists there.

The genitals can best be examined by using a hand-held mirror, and particular attention should be paid to the clitoris. Clients need to start developing sensitivity to touch, which may be something she has carefully avoided. Touching herself, lightly at first, and then sensually, can gradually be developed until it leads to self-stimulation. Some clients may need advice on how to do this. Many books are available on the subject. Piercings of the clitoris, clitoral hood, or labia are recent developments. Some females with any of these piercing report an enhanced sensitivity, others claim it creates a numbness in the area which has led to a frigidity – of the type in which they do not want to be touched in that area. So piercing is another question that can be asked.

ALICIA: Do you have any dynamic treatments for frigidity?

HH: Some people, men as well as women, go through life first creating and then reproducing circumstances in which they are constantly humiliated and rejected. Psychologists call it *secondary* gain. This enables them to wallow in self-pity, seek sympathy from others, and draw attention to themselves, and generally satisfy a part of themselves while greatly dissatisfying another part. They seem, to others, never to learn from each experience, and go through life wreaking vengeance – or at least righteous indignation – on successive partners.

Treatment should initially be counselling, and in

48

some cases that will be enough. Merely having a neutral outsider telling her that sex should not be a negative, hostile, insensitive affair, but should be based on mature feeling, trust and enjoyment, with each partner contributing positively to the other, is often all that is needed.

Sometimes, however, it will be necessary to give much deeper therapy, as in a case that comes to mind: her name is Sarah B, aged 22. I first got her into a state of deep relaxation, and continued:

'Now there is a part of you that want to prevent you from enjoying sex. And there is another part of you that really wants you to be able to enjoy sex. It is the conflict between these two parts that is causing you problems at the moment. In order to overcome this problem, you are going to have to bring harmony instead of conflict to these different parts.

'And the way you are going to do this is simply this: I want you to get in touch with that part of you

49

responsible for preventing you from enjoying sex. And when you are in touch, just indicate that to me so that I will know.

'Okay, Sarah. Now I want you to thank that part for all the good things it has done for you in the past. Preventing you from enjoying sex has obviously served a useful purpose. It isn't necessary for us to know what that purpose was, but it would be very helpful if we could determine if that purpose is still being served usefully. Or has it now become obsolete, having completed it work?'

In the event that the part agrees that no useful purpose is now being served, it can be asked whether it is now prepared to allow the client to enjoy sex in the future. If the answer is positive, then that is the end of the problem, and the unconscious mind can be told that "from this moment on, you are going to be able to start enjoying sex." If, on the other hand, the part of the mind responsible for sex enjoyment insists that a useful purpose is still being served, then continue along the following lines:

'We are glad to know that a useful purpose is still being served because that shows that you are still being protected. But, is it possible, Sarah, for that same purpose to be served in another way? Could it be served in some way that enables you to still be protected and yet allows you to be able to enjoy sex at the same time. [Wait for an indication.] The part may channel its needs into some other function – like wiggling the little finger, for example – or perhaps it could be satisfied by *creating a new part* whose sole object is to satisfy the part preventing sex from being enjoyable.'

Another technique I developed is what I called *Making*

Things Worse To Make Them Better.

Sometimes it is useful to block an intended response in order to release it. Many people quite naturally tend to want what is denied them. The more they are frustrated in satisfying their want, the greater the need becomes. So what starts of as a minor want can, if sufficiently frustrated, quickly become a major want.

This technique is particularly successful when used with *Fantasy Imagery,* in which a client is led into a fantasy in which she enters an ideal erotic situation with someone she feels really attracted to. Every time she seems ready to submit sexually, the therapist must force a resistance. By continually restraining her from responding, her determination to respond normally is built up, and finally consented to.

I used this technique on a patient named Roberta V., aged 28, who had been married but the marriage was annulled because of non-consummation. She told me she'd really wanted to have sex with her husband but just found it impossible to let him touch her. To use her words, 'I froze!' Here's how I handled it:

> 'Well, Roberta, there is only one way that I know that could get you out of the tangle you're in. The trouble is, it wouldn't suit you. I've used it many times before, with great success, but it is only suitable for people who would do what I asked them to do. And in your case, I have to tell you that I don't believe you could. So although the method is virtually guaranteed to work, it's not for you.'

> Obviously, when a carrot like that is held in front of your nose, you'd be pretty annoyed if it wasn't being offered to you. And so it was with Roberta. She couldn't understand why I was so sure she wouldn't be able to do it. I told her because it involved making a promise to my instructions to a 't', and I knew she couldn't do it. The more I told

her this. The more she insisted she could.

That, of course, was part of my plan. By holding it out of her reach, she insisted more and more adamantly that she *would* do whatever I demanded Eventually, when I was sure she meant it, I said I would if she gave me a solemn promise that she would carry out every single thing I told her to do. She promised. Then I continued:

'Okay, Roberta, now I know this isn't going to be easy for you, but believe me, it's the only way. What you are going to do is this: Tonight, at exactly nine o'clock, you are leaving your flat to go to a pub. You are wearing a very thin blouse, see-through, if you have one, and you are not wearing a bra beneath it. If you don't have one, you'll need to go out and buy one. You're wearing a very tight-fitting, very short skirt. And you're not wearing any underwear beneath it. Nothing.

'You're arriving at this pub, you're going inside, and you are taking stock of everyone inside the pub. You're looking for the most *unattractive* man who is sitting alone. You are going across to him and you're sitting down next to him. Then you are leaning close to him and saying the following words: "I'm a virgin and I will pay you fifty pounds to take me to a hotel and fuck me!" If he refuses you are demanding to see the manager of the pub, and you are saying to the manager exactly the following words: "I have offered this man" – pointing to the man – "fifty pounds to take me to a hotel and fuck me. He has refused. I don't think you should allow that kind of person into your pub. Either you ask him to leave or I shall have to leave myself."

'When you have followed these instructions, Roberta, you will be completely cured of your problem. Now don't forget you have promised me you will do it and I shall expect to hear from you tomorrow to that effect.'

Of course, I did hear from Roberta the following morning, exactly as I had anticipated. And it had gone approximately along the lines I thought it would. Roberta had gone home in a state of shell-shock, sat down, and cried her eyes out. Then she had picked up the telephone and called her former husband and begged him to come round to see her, promising to let him have sex with her.

You see, I had given Roberta something to do that I knew she couldn't possibly do. And her only way out, after having given me a solemn promise, was to end her problem. And that's what she did. Her former husband went round to see her, they had made love, and Roberta said that they were going to start seeing each other again, and she hoped they would make everything up. Which I later heard they did.

Of course, Roberta would never have taken that

route if I hadn't made her promise me. And the only way to extract that promise was by leading her into my carefully laid trap: telling her there was a way, but *she* wouldn't be able to do it. If I told her without extracting that solemn promise, she would probably have thought me crazy and walked out of my office, and I might never have heard from her again. And, more than likely, she would still have the problem.

Another special technique I developed was called *Double Indemnity.*

This is a variation of a technique I use frequently for *Ejaculatory Disorders*. With females suffering from frigidity, it can be used in at least two different ways: by females who are unable to attain sexual pleasure due to hostility towards partner, or due to lack of attraction towards partner. Sometimes females fake an orgasm to bring a quick end to their ordeal. I began like this:

'I can fully understand your reasons for that. But what is happening is that you are denying yourself pleasure at the same time. And you don't have to do that! There is a way in which you can pull a fast one over your partner, if that is what you want, and at the same time experience pleasure for yourself without him knowing about it – and thus removing your anxiety about the ordeal.

'When you are going through the motions of faking your orgasm, you can have a *real* orgasm, so he won't know anything about your secret one.'

What the client won't realise is that *you* are pulling a fast one over *her* in the sense that you are merely changing the context of her orgasm. The fake orgasm is all in her mind *and so is the real one!*

If the client is willing to try that, do an Induction, and let client drift into a normal sex scene with her partner, and go through the usual procedure, faking and *actualising* orgasms simultaneously.

Another technique involves the secret, silent orgasm.

> 'I understand that when you don't feel any physical attraction towards a partner it is extremely difficult to show any enthusiasm. But why should you allow him to continue just *using* you without you getting something out of it, too?
>
> 'Well, there is a way in which you can use *him* without him knowing anything about it. It's called the *silent orgasm*. Instead of you subjecting yourself to this selfishness of his, if you set your mind right before you start, so you can be telling yourself all the time that although he thinks he's using *you*, in fact you are the one who is using *him*. And when you're ready, you can lie there as motionless as you like, but you can be having a wonderful, silent

orgasm, made all the sweeter in the knowledge that you are really getting something out of it that he doesn't even know about.'

ALICIA: So you consider frigidity to be a psychological problem?

HH: That's an interesting question because I don't have a total conviction about whether it is psychological or chemical. It might be a bit of both. In the belief that it is psychological, I developed a concept which I called *Sex Reversal*. It goes like this, using kinesiology: Test muscle and say,

'Do I want pleasure?'

'Do I want punishment?'

Obviously, a sexually-healthy person would test strong for the former and weak for the latter. But the female who is *sexually reversed* is different. For them, I would say,

'To deny yourself an orgasm is a form of self-punishment. Obviously, there was a good reason why you felt you deserved punishing – perhaps at an unaware level. It is not important that you or I should know what that reason is. But there comes a time when punishment should cease, when the price has been paid in full. And I want to ask you now, Has your price been paid in full?'

Test muscle. If strong, ask, 'Can I stop punishing myself now, and start to have orgasms?' Test muscle. If strong, that is end of treatment.

If answer to the first question is weak, then follow up with a supplementary question:

'When will my price be paid in full? One week's time? Two week's time?' and so on. Test muscle with each question until getting a strong response.

Or you could say:

'Could the punishment be reduced so that I have an

orgasm on some occasions and not on others?' Test muscle.

If the result of this testing and treatment the problem is brought to an end, as it frequently was, there is a strong case for saying it could be psychological.

MARVIN: I was at a seminar you gave in which you mentioned that there was a sex centre in the brain, but you didn't say what it is. Could you elaborate on it?

HH: I'd love to talk about it. There has always been a big question, Do we have a sex centre in the brain? The answer is Yes, we do! It took a lot of tracking down, like the lymphatic pump, which I discovered in 1992. Except that I found the sex centre much earlier, in 1982. It's quite complicated, so I'll keep it as simple as possible

It is found in area 4 of the Sensorimotor Cortex, known as Brodmann's areas, part of the precentral sulcus of the cerebral cortex). Area 4 contains the *giant Betz cells*, named after Vladamir Betz, a Russian scientist (1834-94), which carry sexual messages from the somatic sensory cortex to the thalamus, where they are converted into *action* or *inaction* by the Betz cells.

These can be located by myoneurologically Test-Pointing (TPing) the left and right *frontal eminences* (FE). The left FE tests for *remembered* experiences, the right FE tests for *constructed* desires. Don't forget we are testing the subject's left side, not the testor's.

So how can we use this information?

2. Test left FE to see if there are any existing barriers that prevent normal sexual expression. If so, correct by tapping 75-100 times to reset optimum levels. Retest.

3. Test right FE to see if you have *erected artificial barriers.* Reasons for this are usually due to problems in left FE. This can be tested by 2-pointing left and right FEs together. If a 2-point changes the muscle indicator

the problem can be corrected by tapping right FE while TPing the left FE, then tapping left FE while TPing right FE.

Some interesting research carried out in the US was done by Dr Beverly Whipple on women who had spinal cord injury and who did not thus experience orgasm. The best they could get was a *phantom orgasm[1]*.

Using PET scans coupled with MRI scans to provide neuroanatomical localisation, and injecting a tracer – horseradish peroxidase – into the wall of the cervix and uterus, she was able to determine the neurological pathways from the Grafenberg or 'G' spot[2] (a sexually sensitive area felt through the vaginal wall) and the clitoris[3].

What she found was that though the normal spinal cord pathways were blocked because of the injury or damage, the tracer was found in cell bodies of the nodose ganglion, which is the sensory ganglion of the vagus nerve, confirming that sensory information was carried via the vagus nerve. Another thing she discovered is that vaginal stimulation caused the release of *vasoactive intestinal peptide* (VIP), a neurotransmitter that acts as a vasodilator that carries messages to the brain via the blood-stream. Similarly, clitoral stimulation causes the release of nitric oxide, which travels in the blood and passes messages to the thalamus.

What's particularly interesting about this, myoneurologically speaking, is that VIP is a neurotransmitter form of the hormone *vasopressin*, also known as *anti-diuretic hormone* (ADH) – manufactured in the posterior pituitary gland. Nitric oxide is formed from arginine as it is broken down by the enzyme *arginase*. And we know we can test for this by TPing Lung 11 (digit 1, medial aspect) on the left side only. If we get a weak muscle which goes strong when we 2-point with the pineal, or a strong muscle that goes weak with the same 2-point, we can say that this is due to a deficiency in the enzyme arginase. We can correct this by tapping L 11 about 25 times. Then retest.

Before trying the correction above we should test for deficiency of *lysine*, which is similar to arginine but without the probability of bringing on a herpes simplex attack. We can test for this at Large Intestine 20 (side of nose) left side only.

JEREMY: You slipped in the term 'phantom orgasm' almost in passing. Can you elaborate on that, and is it anything like the phantom pain that amputees can sometimes get?

HH: I love it when you lot pick me up on what is almost a throwaway line. And that is a very good analogy, Jeremy. There are definite similarities between phantom pain and phantom orgasms. There is an abundance of cases noted in medical literature, many of them relating to horrific accidents – particularly those incurring damage to the spinal cord, pelvis or the genital areas. This is one of those questions which I could either spend a lot of time on or pass it off in a few sentences. Let's see how it develops.

Much to do with orgasms takes place in the brain, and as I've stated earlier, in the Sex Centre[4]. Many females – and males too, actually – have given themselves an orgasm simply by thinking about it intensely. Lady Gaga said in an interview in 2010 that she's enjoyed 'thinking herself off' on numerous occasions. Just as a matter of interest, how many people here have had an orgasm without touching themselves or being touched – in a sexual way – simply by thinking hard about it … willing yourself to have one, if you like? [several hands went up, including a couple of males] Interesting. There is proof, right there, that a phantom orgasm is achievable.

Dr Kenneth Ray Stubbs said he had achieved orgasm through meditation[5] – something he called 'transformative orgasm' and others called 'sacred orgasm'. He described it as something that transcends a normal physical orgasmic experience and becomes a total whole-being, whole-mind orgasm. Those are my words, not his, so I'm paraphrasing him for the sake of brevity. And he encouraged many others, successfully, to achieve the same orgasmic experience. So those were concrete examples of people attaining orgasms purely through thought.

William R Stayton, ThD, PhD, was a Baptist minister, sex therapist and sexuality counsellor. He said that he knew of many people who had had orgasms whilst praying or singing hymns. *'Calling orgasms'* became so named by people in a congregation calling out as they attained orgasm – either to record their achievement or to stimulate others to do the same. I suspect, though I don't have scientific proof, that the intense vibration caused by the singing stimulates those Giant Betz cells we talked about earlier, and that brought on the orgasm. It has been recorded that some opera singers – female – have had orgasms while reaching particularly high notes.

There have been numerous cases recorded of spine-damaged people having an orgasm, sometimes by *willing* it to come, or in other cases by people gently touching another part of the body which was sensitive to touch.

RADINE: You mentioned the G spot. Can you tell us more about it.

HH: The Chinese (and the Indians) have had a very enlightened approach to sex for thousands of years, whereas the Occidentals are approaching enlightenment only in the last 40-50 years. One of the features of their approach is that the female is equally entitled to enjoy sex. Hundreds of techniques were developed to help women achieve their orgasm.

One of their discoveries was the G-spot and the orgasmic epicentre, although the credit is usually attributed

– in the West, anyway – to Dr Stefan Gräfenberg, which I'll come back to. They claim that in order for a female to orgasm there must be a degree of G-spot engorgement. This engorgement can be verified by checking with a finger. The underside of the finger is inserted into the vagina just below the clitoris. The G-spot zone is extruded like an upside-down ridge hanging over the vaginal ceiling.

The epicentre is much deeper inside – too far for a finger to reach, and is placed just above and slightly behind the cervix. They believe that the Orgasmic Wave Energy is pumped out by the contraction of the uterus. The pelvic cavity burns up testosterone which then traps and resonates with the orgasmic waves.

The main acupuncture channel for this is the Ren (Conception Vessel). Ren 2 directly influences the clitoris, which can be stimulated by lightly massaging Ren 2 in a clockwise direction about 25 times. Ren 3 and Ren 4 both stimulate the burning of testosterone in the pelvic cavity, also in a clockwise direction.

Now for the Western version. The Gräfenberg Spot, usually shortened to the G Spot, is a small area – about the size of a small bean – situated on the inner wall of the vagina which is actually the paraurethral gland. It is also called Skene's gland, and has been termed the female prostate. It is about two to three inches inside the vagina, so is easily accessed by fingers, penis or vibrator. But because it is on the front wall of the vagina, that's to say, facing away from a normal penile entry in the missionary position, may not be stimulated in this way. Entry from the rear enables the penis to normally stimulate it with rhythmic strokes, which is why so many women enjoy the 'doggy style' so much. The fingers, of course, can be bent to reach it easily, and vibrators or dildos with curves find it easily accessible. It is highly sensitive to any kind of friction and can certainly enhance the orgasmic sensation. At one time – in the days of Masters & Johnson – it was said that the only orgasm a female could have is a clitoral orgasm. They denied the existence of a vaginal orgasm and even Ernst Gräfenberg, a German gynaecologist, was exploring the possibility of stimulation of the urethra as being more responsible for a female orgasm. He called it a U Spot for that reason.

SARAH: Isn't the U Spot responsible for so-called squirting?

HH: Sort of. The Skene's glands, or paraurethral glands are where the female lubrication is stored and in some females this storage is more developed than in others, which is why some women are able to 'squirt' copious amounts. And just to dispel the myth, squirting has nothing whatever to do with urine, which can only come from the bladder. It is a totally different secretion, although it is often considered to be the same by some people[3].

SARAH: So squirting has nothing to do with the Bartholin's glands?

HH: I won't say it has nothing to do with it. The Bartholin's glands – also known as the greater vestibular glands – have a similar function to Skene's glands – also known as the *lesser* vestibular glands – in that they both help lubricate the vagina. Most experts today believe there are two separate entities: the G Spot[4] (from Graaf's research) and the U-spot (from Skene's glands, or urethral sponge as that area is generally known – and that might include the Bartholin's glands). So the G Spot is responsible for high-energy orgasms and the U-spot for squirting.

Just to make matters even more confusing, there is the A-spot – the *anterior fornix erogenous zone* – also known as the AFE zone or even the 2nd G-spot.

SARAH: Oh, we definitely need to know more about that.

HH: Don't we all! I really don't know much about it myself. It was discovered around 1993 by a Malaysian sex therapist and is located in a small area of the inner ceiling

73

of the vaginal roof. It is stimulated by rapid light tapping of that area and is said to bring a woman to orgasm extremely quickly.

SARAH: If it's too quick we might not enjoy it as much. [laughter]

HH: Ha ha … enjoyment is a personal thing. I haven't even mentioned the rectouterine pouch, sometimes called the Douglas Pouch.

SARAH: Wow! Does that give longer-lasting orgasms? [more laughter]

HH: Maybe, for some. If you think of the AFE being the anterior of the anterior fornix, then the Douglas Pouch is the *posterior* equivalent.

JACK: I heard somewhere that some women's clitoris is in a constant state of erection? Is that true, and if it is, does this affect the female in any adverse way?

HH: It is true, it's called clitorism, and it can be quite painful for them. In a way, it is similar to priapism in some males, except that in their case because the penis is so much larger than the clitoris it is more difficult to conceal and can cause huge embarrassment. In the case of females, it's not so much embarrassment as discomfort in many cases. While some women complain of pain attached to the condition, others have claimed that it has enhanced their sexual appetite to the point where they can never get enough sex … and by sex, they mean clitoral-stimulation sex.

JACK: Does that mean that all nymphomaniacs have this clitorism?

HH: No, separate problem, although that's not to say some nymphomaniacs don't also have clitorism. Actually, Jack, the term 'nymphomania' is no longer used … I don't know whether it's considered not politically correct or whatever, but the preferred term now is *hypersexuality*, which for men was previously called satyriasis. Dr Candace Pert claimed that research on animals showed that hyperactive sex activity showed a 200% increase of endorphins in the blood supply.

Endorphins are *opioid neuropeptides* produced in the pituitary gland and the hypothalamus. The endorphins produced in the pituitary – *ß-endorphins* – are released into the bloodstream, while those produced in the hypothalamus are released in the spinal cord and brain. Around 1992, two other scientists – Czech analytical chemist Lumír Ondřej Hanuš and American molecular pharmacologist William Anthony Devane – discovered another brain chemical, *anandamide*[5], which, if proved to be in excess, might supply the missing link between those people, male and female, who have a 'normal' sex desire and those who have an excessively high sex desire. What this means is that it might turn out that hypersexuality, which was thought to be a purely psychological problem, might well prove to be a biochemical one. I find it most interesting that so many things, that have for so long been considered to be psychological in origin, are being discovered to be of a chemical nature. This, of course, adds ammunition to those who say there is no such thing as the mind. If we extend that, could it be that there is no such thing as *imagination*? That, too, is a series of chemical reactions within the body or brain?

FRED: Isn't our imagination tied in with our personal belief system?

HH: That is such a terrific question I don't know if you fully appreciate the significance of it.

FRED: [shrugging] I was only thinking aloud.

HH: Well, I'm going to tell you why it is such a good question, because it cuts right through to the very existence of matter through our understanding of quantum physics. Candace Pert's *The Molecules of Emotion* was followed up by another book she wrote called *The Physics of Emotion*. In it, she explains how vibrating energy is the source of everything – including emotions. Just going back to the earlier part of the 20ᵗʰ Century, argument raged between proponents of Einstein's theory of energy being in the form of particles and Thomas Young who claimed all energy came in the form of waves. Then in the 1920s along came Niels Bohr who said that energy could be in the form of waves *and* particles. This argument plunged the scientific community into crisis, and in 1927 Bohr and several other leading scientists and 'thinkers' came together and came up with what became known as the Copenhagen Interpretation, which said this: (my own words) energy is a pure wave form *until* concentration, thought or focus is put on it, causing the wave form to collapse and form a particle or particles. And the thought or focus that an individual puts on something exists because of our belief system.

FRED: I'm not quite following this, Harry. This table I'm sitting at is still a table, whether I think it is or not. I know it's all made up from billions of atoms which are all moving and vibrating but their density gives us the impression of being solid.

HH: Okay, you see it as a table. Probably everyone sitting in this hall see it as a table. But a tribesman in the Kalahari might see it as a piece of wood for the fire. That thought has more practicality to him. A minister of the church might see lead guttering on the church roof as guttering; someone else might see it as scrap metal that could be stolen and sold for a profit. You see, it is our perception of something that gives it reality. Everything around us in the world outside our body is interpreted through our senses. The information from outside us comes in the form of waves and our brain interprets those waves into something we can make sense of. And that will be the result of previous experiences we have had – together with communication with others who aid our learning experience. Others teach us that that piece of wood is a table and that is what we recognise it as. But the Kalahari tribesman doesn't encounter a table like that, so he doesn't recognise it as such.

Let me give you another example. During Charles Darwin's adventures in the Beagle, he called at the Galápagos Archipeligo in the Pacific Ocean. The islanders rowed their canoes out to greet Darwin's boat which was being rowed towards the shore. What's amazing is that the islanders saw the ship's boat but they didn't see the Beagle – *because they had never seen a big sailing ship before. It was outside their experience.* Of course, when many of them were later taken out to the ship they then saw it. And it became a part of their belief system thereafter.

I can give you other examples. A scientist did some experiments with fleas. He put a sheet of glass about four inches from the floor. When the fleas kept jumping up they would bang their heads on the glass, so very quickly they learnt not to jump as high as four inches. Later, when the glass was removed, the fleas continued to jump just below four inches and never above it. In a somewhat similar experiment, a scientist placed a sheet of glass in the centre of a tank containing goldfish on both sides of the glass. When they started banging their heads against the glass – which, of course, they couldn't see – they would only swim just short of the glass and then turn round again. When later the glass was removed, the goldfish on both sides of the tank would only swim as far as the glass had been and would then turn back. None of the goldfish would swim beyond where the glass had been placed. Their belief systems led them to believe the glass was still there.

One final example, which I saw in Sri Lanka, at the famous Elephant's Orphanage at Pinnawela. At night, the young elephants are tethered to a post by a few feet of thin rope, which they could very easily snap if they tried to. But they don't try. When they are first brought to the Orphanage, they are tethered by a strong chain, which they could not break. Once they have become accustomed to the chain it is changed for a rope because the keepers know the elephants will not attempt to break free. Their belief system has been established.

FRED: I'm beginning to see the real significance of what you're saying. What is staggering is that it took humans literally thousands of years to understand this.

HH: And we're getting the benefit of those peoples experience which enables us to think ahead to how we can apply it in our own lives. I was once giving a course in hypnosis – I see a few faces of people who were at the course in question – and I held up a piece of plain white paper. I should add that none of the people were at the time in a hypnotic state. I got them to concentrate on the piece of paper, then I suddenly crumpled it up and threw it to the ground. I think I might ask Jennie to tell you what happened.

JENNIE: Oh God, yes. I remember several people just flaked out. There were literally about a dozen people slumped on the floor totally out of it. One guy, sitting close to me, just sat there crying and bawling. Now this was a big bruiser-type guy, a real hard case. And to see him sitting crying was kind of blowing my mind. I remember rushing over to Harry and telling him to come quickly to do something for the guy.

DELIA: I was there that day and I thought we needed to send for some ambulances. I seem to remember the only person who didn't seem perturbed was Harry.

HH: Well, I'd done it before with other groups, so I knew what to expect. I knew that out of fifty to sixty people there were going to be a few who would react in this way. These were all people who had serious self-esteem problems. When I crumpled the paper, which they associated themselves with, they saw it as their whole personality being crushed. It was a rather cruel way to sort out a few people I could work with to help them overcome their problem. It might have seemed bad at the time but every one of them benefited very quickly.

JENNIE: Changing the subject quickly, Harry, you mentioned the use of vibrators along with the G Spot and I'm wondering if there are any hidden dangers attached to vibrators?

HH: I'm glad you asked that otherwise it might have slipped away unnoticed. What most people don't know is whether or not vibrators can actually cause damage. And the answer is yes. Here's what they can do:

- it abrades the clitoral and G-spot nerves and tissue

- can also damage the urethral and bladder's parasympathetic nerves that control urinary incontinence, resulting in urethral female ejaculation.

The use of vibrators, biking and horse-riding, can all damage the superficial nerves of the clitoris and labia. This can affect arousal normally leading to an orgasm, and cause a fall-back on G-spot and Epicentre orgasm – which is a different kind of orgasm. [Can use **Clitoroil** treatment]

Orgasm physically depends on the ratio between testosterone and oestrogen. With friction (through masturbation or intercourse), testosterone becomes electrically charged and heats the clitoral and pudendal nerves when it is burned and converted to *dihydrotestosterone* (DHT). Oestrogen cools the nerves (like a water-cooling system), which causes them to discharge – creating the Orgasmic Wave. Too much oestrogen has the effect of over-cooling the process (going off the boil, so to speak), and can also lead to thickening of the tissue thickness surrounding the G-spot, thus reducing sexual stimulation to that point.

Women with high oestrogen levels should be stimulated at the Epicentre, which is equivalent to the male prostate. Stimulating the Epicentre with a rhythmic pressure of about 1 KSC (kilos per square centimetre) can trigger an orgasm even when oestrogen levels are very high.

That is why labour can give women an orgasm providing there is no significant pain.

The best treatment I can suggest is the homeopathic HH 960 Clitostore, which is specifically designed to repair damage to the clitoris and soft vaginal tissue (including the G-spot).

BRENDA: You've talked about Dyspareunia but you haven't really said anything about vaginismus.

HH: Yes, that's partly because you lot jump from one thing to another before I've really finished on a subject. Vaginismus is a severe contraction of vaginal muscles prior to penetration, usually causing considerable pain and chronic tension.

Primary vaginismus is organic in origin, while *Secondary vaginismus* has a psychogenic basis. It is essential to have a physical examination before treatment can be planned. Physical factors could include:

- Congenital deformation of the vagina

- Introital damage or infection (to entrance of vagina)

- Retroversion of the uterus

- Pelvic tumour

- Polyps

- Cervicitis (inflammation of the cervix uteri . neck of the uterus)

- Tender episiotomy scar (surgical incision in vulva for obstetric purposes)

- Kraurosis vulvae (dry glistening condition of the mucous membrane of the vulva, characterised by intense itching and constitutional disturbance from loss of sleep)

- Urethral caruncle (small bright red growth at entrance of the urethra. It is very painful, and bleeds readily on being touched)

Despite this list of organic causes, most cases of vaginismus are psychogenic, and commonly include any of the following:

- Faulty psychosexual development

- Fear of being too small

- Defence against contraception, often due to religious convictions)

- Hostility against partner

- Phobic reaction to penetration by a foreign object

- Fear of pregnancy

- Reaction to partner having a sexual dysfunction mother's command (as a child) to always keep her legs crossed

There is often a strong secondary gain, with the client wanting to be helped, yet at the same time being frightened because once cured she no longer has a defence against intercourse, which is what she fears. In some cases, it is possible to trace the condition to a single frightening experience, which thus created a phobic condition.

Partners frequently need treatment themselves as there is a tendency for a man to develop secondary impotence as a direct result of his partner's vaginismus.

Counselling is often a good first step in treatment, especially when there is a need to correct faulty conceptions, i.e. religious misconceptions, Victorian-style upbringing – 'Close your eyes and think of Jesus' – or childhood fears of sex.

I have found in practice that a frequent factor causing vaginismus is the result of indecent exposure by an adult man to a young girl, in which what seems to her like an enormous penis. Quite naturally, when the girl learns – if she doesn't already know – that intercourse is penile entry to her vagina, it is not surprising that she finds it a frightening proposition.

Counselling for that kind of belief/fear usually needs to be followed up by something more powerful than just counselling; indeed, a female might not be conscious of the reason. Sometimes, an extremely painful introduction to sex might create a phobic anxiety, in which she believes that all sex will be as painful as that first time.

Vaginismus may be employed as a defence against having to endure intercourse, or it might be a way of demonstrating hostility towards partner. Either case should show up through the questionnaire and in either case a strategy of treatment can be prepared.

Linchpinning

This is a technique I developed for *Myoneurology* but in this case we are going to use it in a different manner. [A *linchpin* is to lightly squeeze the Chinese pulse area of the left wrist at the appropriate time – when you want to link it with a person's experience as a future reminder] A simple method of dealing with a phobic anxiety is not merely to take it away – the client might well have a psychological need for it – but to offer another choice, or choices.

Let's take an example:

Maria has vaginal spasms because she has a terrible fear of being penetrated by a foreign object, i.e. penis. Now, instead of removing the fear of penises altogether, after inducing a light trance we can say:

> 'And you are finding, Maria, that whenever you are in a situation of facing sexual intercourse with a man whose penis is at least 30 cm long – **linchpin** – you are experiencing painful vaginal spasms, and intercourse is becoming impossible. But on all other occasions – **linchpin** – when your partner has a penis of less than 30 cm, there is no need for you to feel any painful spasms at all. In fact, you are finding yourself capable of really enjoying sex –

linchpin – with a partner whose penis is less than 30 cm long.'

Laying the first linchpin establishes a time when the vaginal spasms she has already been encountering may return. And since our 30 cm man is so remote, the anxiety is never likely to return. Remember that a phobic anxiety is only a learned response that is aroused whenever confronted with a particular stimuli. Whenever that stimulus is presented the response is always the same. We additionally linchpin the other two *overwhelming* linchpins that on all other occasions she is going to find intercourse pleasurable.

Changing Memory

One of the great things about people with phobic anxieties is that they're easy to treat. The reason they're easy to treat is that they're easy to influence. The very fact that they have a phobic response to a set stimuli pattern is proof of that. The vast majority of us can't achieve that, which means that we're not so easy to influence. So when we get clients who say that they always respond in the same way to the same stimuli, i.e. painful vaginal spasms, we know that it should not be difficult to change that response.

Linchpinning is one way, Changing Memory is another, more subtle way. We want to get the client onto her time line:

'So which direction is the future [wait for her to point] and which direction is the past [wait for her to point]. Okay, Maria, and I want you to go back in time to the very first occasion when you experienced those painful spasms. Go all the way back, and I shall be going back with you. So you'll still hear my voice and be aware of my presence, but you will be there in mind and in body, exactly as it was then. And you will hear my voice throughout and will know I am there with you, to help keep you safe and secure. You can see everything the way it was. Nod your head when you are there. [When client nods, test muscle. Should be weak]

'Will you tell me where you are and who you are with? [wait] Can you describe in detail what happened? [wait]

'Okay. Now I want you to go through all that again, except that this time, instead of being there, I want you to stand outside the experience – above your time line – and *watch yourself* undergoing that experience once again.

'And while you're watching it, I want you to realise that there is something about yourself that you know but you don't know that you know. And as soon as you find out what it is you know but don't know that you know, you can find the whole experience becomes pleasant and enjoyable. And when it's finished, please nod. [Wait, then test muscle. Should now be strong]

'Now Maria, can you tell me what happened when you were watching yourself?' [wait]

If the experience was a pleasant one, as suggested, then bring client forward, and let her experience *in imaginal* having sex with her normal partner. If the experience was a repeat of the former, unpleasant one, continue as follows:

'And as you return to the present, here with me now, part of your mind will still be considering what it is that you know but don't know that you know, in relation to that former painful experience. And as soon as it becomes available to your conscious mind, you will become aware of it, and from that moment on you will be able to respond normally and without any further painful vaginal spasms in the future.'

It might take hours, days or weeks for the deeply hidden information to filter its way through to the client's awareness.

<u>Changing the answer</u>

A simple, but sometimes effective method is to ask the client to go deep inside herself and ask the question,

'Why does your vagina keep saying no?'

Wait for an answer. Then ask,

'What would happen if your vagina said yes?'

How you respond will depend on the answer she gives.

For Vaginismus, as for other forms of sexual dysfunction, we have a specially designed questionnaire:

Questionnaire

<u>Beliefs</u>

1.   do you have any strong religious beliefs?

2.   do you have any strong religious beliefs about sex?

3.   do you believe that a man should dominate sexually?

4.   do you believe that it is a woman's duty to please her partner sexually?

Relationships

1.   how would you describe your relationship with your partner?

2.   has there been any time in the past when the relationship was

    a)   satisfactory

    b)   good

    c)   really good

    d)   perfect?

3.   is there a part of your relationship that frightens you?

4.   have you ever felt hostility towards your partner? Describe

5.   has your partner at any time had any kind of sexual disorder?

Sexual Relationships

1.   are there any aspects of sex that you find pleasurable?

2.   do you mind being touched by your partner?

3.   do you place any limitations on your partner (i.e. certain parts of the body he may not touch)?

4.   does your partner place any limitations on you?

5.   is your partner very demanding sexually?

6.   do you sometimes/often find yourself compelled to enter into sex without your approval?

7.   what would happen if you refused?

8.   has your partner tried means other than intercourse to bring sexual pleasure to you? Describe

9.   have you tried means other than intercourse to bring sexual pleasure to your partner? Describe

Upbringing

1. were you brought up strictly?

2. what was your mother's attitude towards sex?

3. what was your father's attitude towards sex?

4. when you were a child, did anything happen to frighten you sexually?

5. how would you describe your relationship with your mother?

6. how would you describe your relationship with your father?

7. what sort of relationship did you have with brothers/sisters?

Body Image

1. what do you think of your hair? Style, texture, colour, etc?

2. how about your eyes?

3.   nose. Are you satisfied with it? Would you like it changed in any way?

4.   how about your mouth? Are you satisfied with it?

5.   voice. How do you feel about your voice?

6.   what about your arms?

7.   how about your hands?

8.   your overall figure. What do you think about it? Height, weight, etc.?

9.   how about your breasts? Are they too big, too small, too saggy?

10. and the nipples. Are they too dark, too small, too big?

11. how about your stomach? How do you feel about your stomach?

12. and how about your hips?

13. genitals. How do you feel about your genitals?

14. do you ever feel that your vagina is too tight, too small?

15. what about your buttocks? Satisfied?

16. what about your thighs? How do you feel about your thighs?

17. legs?

18. feet? Satisfied or not satisfied with your feet?

19. how about your personality? How do you feel about that?

20. how do you feel about your partner's body? Are there any parts that frighten or disgust you? Describe

Outline of Dysfunctions

1. under what circumstances have you experienced an orgasm, if ever?

2. do you prefer masturbation to intercourse?

3. have you ever had a happy sex relationship other than with present partner?

4. at what point did you first experience vaginismus?

5.   how does your partner generally respond to your

discomfort? Does he understand and try to be gentle?

Does he get angry or violent?

GERRY: Can I change the subject completely and ask

about oral sex? Are there any risks attached to it?

HH: I presume you are talking about fellatio, and

whether there are risks for the female?

GERRY: I was asking about any kind of oral sex,

including cunnilingus between male and female or female

to female.

HH: Oh, okay. Let's take the female on male first –

fellatio. There is the obvious danger of sexually transmitted

disease. There isn't normally too much risk, but if there are

any lesions, scratches, ulcers or cuts in the mouth or lips

there is a much higher element of risk of infection. There is

always a possibility of transmitting Aids from a carrier

although this is not frequently a cause. The dangers of anal intercourse are greater in this respect. Gonorrhoea, syphilis and Chlamydia can all be sexually transmitted during oral sex, especially from fellatio. Rimming – that's oro-anal contact for those who don't know the term or the practice – carries a far greater risk of STD, including Hepatitis A, B and C and in particular, worms.

So far as cunnilingus is concerned, the same elements are possible as just described but at a reduced level of risk – except in the case of rimming, where it remains equally high in both genders.

MARK: As an ignorant male – well, maybe not *that* ignorant – who always hopes that his partner is going to have an orgasm, could you tell us something about the technicalities of a female orgasm?

HH: Okay. I can understand that males have the disadvantage of not always knowing if their partner has had an orgasm or not because of the female's ability to 'fake' an orgasm. Not only that but many if not most females can have multiple orgasms, something which is comparatively rare amongst males. So it can come down to libido – is the female's libido sufficiently aroused? – or technique – is enough time spent on foreplay, and is the foreplay adequately stimulating? – or any of a wide range of other factors that can orgasmic difficulties in a female.

The main hormone for libido in both males and females is *testosterone,* the male sex hormone, but also produced in the female adrenal glands. The amino acid *tyrosine* is a precursor for *dopamine*, which stimulates the libido. We can use Myoneurology to check for levels of dopamine, as follows: The TP for tyrosine is found at the lateral aspect of the 1st phalange of the fourth (ring) finger – SJ 1 in acupuncture. *Phenylalalanine* is another amino acid which is converted into a neurotransmitter of the same name. This is a relaxant, but also helps deal with stress and agitation. So if the problem can be helped by relieving stress this might help, and can be tested for and stimulated myoneurologically. The TP is found at the lateral corner of the eyebrow (there is a small niche there) – GB 1 in acupuncture.

Female orgasms come about initially through mental processes. This is confirmed by the fact that females can have orgasmic dreams, hallucinations, during which time there might be no touching of the genitals. Generally speaking, orgasms do not just happen. Achieving them is a learning process, and if a female is unable to achieve them it is usually because they she not learned a suitable technique for doing so.

It also requires concentration, of course. If a female is thinking about what to cook for dinner, or whether she has to do the washing-up afterwards, it could be difficult to achieve orgasm. Worse if she is thinking that perhaps her partner is being, or has been, unfaithful towards her, or if she fears his anger or even violence.

I always try to get patients to condition their mind

for every important occasion. It can become a habit, and when it does things work much more efficiently. Sometimes it is necessary to give direct information about the physiological functions of the female genitals. Some females are so mentally dissociated from their body that they don't even know that they can derive much pleasure through manipulation of the clitoris. Because a female client can be too embarrassed discussing masturbation for *herself*, a useful technique is to talk about it indirectly:

'This is surprisingly common among young men. Perhaps they've been brought up to believe that even touching the genitals is a sin. As a result, they don't know *how* to achieve an orgasm through masturbation . And yet they do have orgasms through dreams.

'And sometimes they are aware of their penis becoming semi-erect, and then fully erect, and they aren't aware of what it can mean, or what they might do. And then I tell them that it is all right for them to stimulate themselves manually to orgasm. And it comes as a tremendous relief for them to discover that masturbation is as natural as breathing and eating.

'And we are all half male and half female, anyway. And anything that a male can achieve so a female can achieve. As males can commonly have orgasms through dreams, so can females.

'And as tumescence occurs in the male penis when he becomes sexually aroused, so it also occurs in the female clitoris when she becomes aroused. And as a man can stimulate his penis until he achieves orgasm, so can a female stimulate her clitoris.

'The wonderful thing about masturbation is that it is Nature's way of allowing us to learn how to prepare ourselves for the sex act with others. When they have learnt how to achieve orgasm, some people, males and females, gradually cease to masturbate. Others prefer to retain this practice. It doesn't really matter.'

Change of Motivation

Some prostitutes and some nymphomaniacs find it difficult or even impossible to achieve an orgasm. The reasons here are quite different from other cases, the first using sex merely as a means of exploitation, the latter in a fruitless search for a satisfaction which is never achieved.

To change either of these types requires a *change of motivation*. Clearly there is a conflict of requirements otherwise they would not be coming for treatment. On the one hand they want to achieve an orgasm; on the other, they want to exploit men, either for money for an unrealistic ideal. And what they are doing is completely incongruous: they are having plenty of sex and they are not enjoying it one little bit. It is not a question of techniques because both types probably know more about various techniques than do any of us. It is a question of mind set: they are indulging in sex, not for pleasure, but for another reason which has nothing to do with pleasure.

It is important here to work at a level *beneath awareness* because they have already demonstrated that awareness exacerbates the problem rather than ameliorating it. Working beneath awareness can be done *metaphorically*:

'Go back in time, way back to the time when you were a very small child. So small that you could only crawl along the floor. You could see other, bigger people walking in the room but you could still only crawl. And you made up your mind that you were going to walk, too.

'But first you had to be able to stand. So you tried to stand, by first pulling yourself up the leg of a chair, falling down several times in the early stages until finally you could do it, not only when holding on to something but even without using your hands at all.

'And then you took your first step. And came crashing down with a bump. But it didn't deter you, and you pulled yourself up again, stood up, and took another step, tentatively. You fell down again.

'But as you repeated this over and over again you managed to go from one step to two, and from two steps to three, until you were walking all around the room without falling once.

'You became so good at it that before long you were able to walk and run without even having to look down at your feet to make sure you were going in the right direction. You could climb stairs and you could go down stairs without any difficult at all.

'And a few years later you went to school. You'd noticed that grown-ups, and even a lot of other children, could pick up a book and all the little things that were written on a page seemed to make sense to them. They called it reading. And you wanted to learn to read. But first you had to learn what all the little letters meant.

'At first it made no sense at all to you. How could you tell the difference between a p and a q? You thought you'd never learn it, but you were determined, because the *rewards were worthwhile*.

'So you struggled on until eventually it all clicked into place. And the same with reading. You wanted to learn to read, to turn all those words into sounds, and although it was a struggle you made it.

'Now, today, you have no difficult in walking, or reading. You don't have to watch each foot as you come down the stairs. In fact, if you tried you'd be more likely to stumble over your feet. And when you're reading, you don't have to study each letter that makes up a word. You just read in chunks of letters and perhaps even in chunks of words.

'You did all these things, despite the difficulties, because you wanted to. You wanted to be able to do things that other people seem to take for granted. Things that added to the quality of life and to the pleasures of life.

'Yet in a strange and curious way, you never quite managed to master the pleasures of sex. You know, when we read a book written in our own language, we read across the page from left to right. Yet the Chinese read from right to left. Think what would have happened if we tried to read our books as the Chinese read theirs. It wouldn't make any sense to us.

'But there are people, in this country, who actually try to read a book from right to left, because that is the way they decided to learn. As a result, they can't make any sense out of a page and they *can't get any real pleasure* from reading a book.

'These people are actually quite intelligent, and there is a part of them that actually knows they are *depriving themselves of pleasure*, yet they might not know why.

'Perhaps they are *afraid* of something. Yet they have no need to be afraid of something which *comes naturally* for most people.... '

There is a combination of learning behaviour, motivation,

and metaphorical change in that example. I always make a point of not trying to explain meanings to a client when doing metaphorical work. It is important that their own mind should evaluate and extract any meaningful phrases and apply it.

We do have a questionnaire available, which is going to be handed out now. [For the benefit of readers it is reproduced below]

Questionnaire

Outline of Dysfunction

1.   Have you at any time achieved an orgasm?

2.   At what point were you unable to achieve orgasm through intercourse?

3.   Can you attain orgasm now through masturbation?

4.   Do you sometimes indicate to partner that you have had an orgasm even when you have not?

5.   Are you able to achieve an orgasm in some situations

114

and not in others?

6.   What seems to prevent you from having an orgasm?

7.   Does your partner show concern when you do not
     have an orgasm?

8.   Are you afraid to 'let yourself go'?

9.   Are you able to discuss any problems or difficulties
     with partner?

10. Do you and your partner indulge in sexual foreplay?

Upbringing and Childhood

1.   Were you brought up with strong religious
     convictions?

2.   Do you have strong religious convictions now?

3.   Do you have any convictions that *sex* is either bad or
     dirty, and should only be indulged in for procreative
     purposes?

4.   Were you brought up strictly by parents?

5.   Did your mother ever talk to you about sex?

6.   Where and when did you first learn about masturbation?

7.   Were you ever warned against masturbation? By whom?

8.   Were you ever caught indulging in any sexual activity as a child?

Sexual Learning

1.   How did you first learn about sexual intercourse?

2.   What was your initial reaction?

3.   In masturbation do you use your fingers or some object?

4.   Have you tried using a vibrator? Does this help?

5.   Do you like your partner to touch your genitals?

6.   Are you able to communicate openly with partner about your sexual likes and dislikes?

7. Is your partner sometimes/often/never able to bring you to orgasm through (a) coitus (b) manual manipulation (c) oral stimulation

8. Describe a typical sex encounter with partner:

Pregnancy

1. Do you or your partner take contraceptive precautions?

2. Have you had an abortion or miscarriage?

3. Do you worry about becoming pregnant?

4. Does your partner worry about you becoming pregnant?

5. Has your sexual attitude changed as a result of pregnancy?

Relationships

1. Are you still sexually attracted towards partner?

2. Were you ever sexually attracted towards partner?

3.   At what point did your attraction change?

4.   Do you trust your partner?

5.   Are you satisfied that your partner stimulates you adequately?

6.   Are you afraid of your partner in any way?

7.   Has your partner tried to help you to orgasm other than intercourse? Describe:

There is another treatment that I found very effective, which I call

Self-Punishment and Sexual Reversal

Begin by testing any strong muscle and saying – and the patient is asked to repeat it after me as I test the muscle while doing so –

'Do I want pleasure?'

pause

'Do I want punishment?'

Obviously, a sexually-healthy person would test strong for the former and weak for the latter. But the female who is *sexually reversed* is different.

Say:

'To deny yourself an orgasm is a form of self-punishment. Obviously, there was a good reason why you felt you deserved punishing – perhaps at an unaware level. It is not important that you or I should know what that reason is. But there comes a time when punishment should cease, when the price has been paid in full. And I want to ask you now,

Has your price been paid in full?'

Test muscle. If strong, ask, 'Can I stop punishing myself now, and start to have orgasms?' Test muscle. If strong, that is end of treatment.

If answer to the first question is weak, then follow

up with a supplementary question:

'When will my price be paid in full? One week's time? Two week's time?' and so on. Test muscle with each question until getting a strong response.

Or you could say, 'Could the punishment be reduced so that I have an orgasm on some occasions and not on others?' Test muscle.

One last thing on the question of orgasmic difficulty: the role of breathing. The Chinese, in their wisdom, recognised that breathing not only creates a relaxation of mind it also energises the whole body. They developed a rhythmic exercise which has been modified over the centuries and has reached us in the present day in what has become known as Kegel exercises. But the Chinese called it *Qi-Gong Breathing*

This is a method which can help power the brain's

acetylcholine, dopamine and serotonin nervous functions with the essential hormones and nutrients. The acetylcholine and PNS functions are responsible for the promotion of penile/G-spot/clitoral erection and sizes (due to release of 2nd neurotransmitter Nitric Oxide and the arterial dilator cGMP (cyclic Guanosine monophosphate) and mutually associated with the local secretion of the relaxant hormone prostaglandin E-1 (PG-E1) in the local tissues and arterial walls for arterial dilation during lovemaking, in conjunction with the biological action of testosterone and DHEA in the hormone receptors in the brain and sex organs.

The autorhythmic fibres of the Epicentre (the orgasmic pacemaker) are ignited when the dopamine/SNS circuits are bioelectrically triggered by the over-erection (over-stress) of the urethral spongy tissues and nerves in synchronising with the sudden surge of oxytocin released from the pituitary.

If you have a proper erection of the urethral/vaginal spongy tissues, an intensified stimulation will signal the pituitary to release a burst of orgasmic hormone oxytocin, the brain will switch the autonomic nervous function from parasympathetic erection to sympathetic orgasm, and at the same time, the dopamine-norepinephrine-epinephrine (stress hormone) will burst.

Thus, the ultimate uterine/vaginal contraction will be initiated by the orgasmic pacemaker and the orgasmic wave energy will be radiated out of the pelvic cavity, running up to the heart, lungs, forehead, and then the brain's cerebral cortex (your conscious controller) via the frontal energy path (Ren or Conception Vessel of the acupuncture network) so that you will lose conscious control of your body and your heavy breathing, crying, moaning, and movement of body parts are synchronising with the 0.8 seconds beating rate of the uterine/vaginal contraction.

This whole process can be totally enhanced by what I call the Qi-Gong Breathing Cycle. Exerting an inhaling (qi) pressure against the bladder is to turn the bladder's sensory-parasympathetic nervous circuits for over-riding the prostate/uterine sensory-sympathetic (ejaculation and orgasmic) circuits. So does contracting the coccyx.

The bioelectric recharge is done by burning testosterone in the local tissues. The pelvic cavity is the normal hormone reception centre. The tissues contain a lot of testosterone and oestrogen receptors that can trap a lot of testosterone and oestrogen respectively. The Epicentre (the area between prostate and bladder in men and between cervix and bladder in women) is the testosterone reception centre. Burning testosterone there promotes libido and drives orgasm high during sexual activity.

During this Qi Gong Breathing Exercise, the bladder's PNS nerves discharge bioelectric flow into the Ren circuit, and when you are contracting the coccygeal muscle the bioelectric flow moves across the anus from CV-1 (between the anus and scrotum or between anus and vagina) to Du-1, where the bioelectric energy partially flows into the Du channel and partially feeds the sensory nerves around the coccyx.

Then the bioelectric current in the sensory nerves is split into two parts in the inter-neuron switches-splitters inside the S-1 to S-5 and Coccyx. A large part of energy is coupled in the spinal cord nerves/CNS to the brain's cerebral cortex (sensory and then motor areas for response; the rest of the energy is reflected back to the genital area through the S-1 to S-5 and CO parasympathetic motor nerves that drive the erection and engorgement blood pressures from the pubis-penis (clitoris and vaginal/urethral spongy tissues) groins to the coccyx. This means you activate the orgasmic/ejaculation circuits.

The Exercise

Think about having an orgasm-ejaculation.

Test muscle. May be weak.

Contract coccygeal muscle during the in-breath and relax during out-breath.

Do 3 cycles, then test muscle.

GERALDINE: Could you say something about birth control? There are so many different methods available today and a lot of questions have been asked about the Pill, but what about the day-after pill? And the one where you have only two or three injections a year.

HH: What a terrific question. And it's something I completely left out of my introductory talk –and should have put in. You're absolutely right, there are quite a lot of hazards attached to some of these pills. Just as a matter of interest, are there any Catholics here who use pregnancy prevention methods … don't feel obliged to put your hand up if you prefer to keep it personal but it would be interesting to see how many are acting against their religious beliefs. [about a dozen hands go up, all female] And just as added interest, are there any who do abide by birth control for moral or religious reasons? [two hands go up]. Interesting. I don't want to make a thing about that because it is not my place to do so but statistically, in this hall anyway, there are about five or six times as many females who are making their own decisions rather than having them made for them.

Okay, as for the use of the Pill, first of all there are so many different types that it is difficult to generalise. The medical profession recognises this by the very fact that they frequently change one pill for another, according to symptoms which might develop. Also, some pills suit some females more than others. There is no one pill which suits everybody. But the one thing they all have in common is that they do disrupt or interfere with a female's natural menstrual cycle. They override the normal cycle. This can cause the hypothalamus, the pituitary or the ovary to stop – or at least moderate – the normal production of female hormones. When a female later decides she wants to have a child and stops taking the Pill, she might find that she has reproductive difficulties. Not only that but they can cause bloating, liver damage – even cancer – severe PMS – and breast problems.

The morning-after pill is something of a misnomer because it works for up to three days after intercourse. There is a new one on the market called *Ellaone* that works for up to five days. Their main use is for females who have had unprotected sex, have had a condom burst during sex, or have been the victims of rape. Not enough hard evidence is yet available to say what all the pros and cons are. All I would say is that should be used only as a real emergency.

The other part of Geraldine's question is the really interesting one. The one where three injections are given. The substance commonly used is Depo Provera. Women are always told that it's perfectly safe, but look at these side effects, already experienced by a growing number of women:

1. up to 25 kilos weight gain – that's more than 55 pounds

2. extreme excitability, nervousness

3. panic attacks, paranoia

4. shortness of breath

5. great loss of libido

6. painful intercourse

7. severe lack of lubrication

8. lowered immune system

9. loss of hair

10. unwanted hair on breasts, toes, face

11. violent headaches

12. extremely sore, stiff muscles all over body

13. blurry vision

14. dizziness

15. inability to bend over

16. severe neck and shoulder pain

17. breast tenderness and pains

18. heart palpitations

19. chronic sinus and yeast infections

20. concentration and memory problems

21. acne

22. suicidal thoughts because daily debilitating pain too
    much to bear

Now let's take a look at what happens when you start

having these shots. Progestin (a pseudo-progesterone)

poisons the liver, disables the ovarian functions, negatively

disturbs the brain's dopamine, acetylcholine nervous

systems and slows down thyroid functions, resulting in mood-swings, depression, weight gain, vaginal dryness, intercourse or penetration pain, loss of libido, breast tenderness, tiredness, fatigue, joint pains, muscular cramps, blurry vision, dizziness, yeast infection, immune weakness, headaches, menstrual interruption and so on. All the symptoms reported above.

Generally, birth control shots or implants produce more and broader damage than the pills do (and they're bad enough!). The common problems of the birth control drugs are the increasing production of prolactin (a hormone made in the pituitary gland, which inhibits orgasms) and the decreasing production of dopamine and testosterone due to the poisoned liver. The liver has to deactivate all the other functions and to work extremely hard to detoxify this toxin.

Here's how progestin works: It binds into the progesterone receptors to trigger the brain's Progesterone Negative Feedback Controller in the hypothalamus-pituitary-ovarian axis, and refuses to go away once it takes over the receptors. Its behaviours are like street drugs, but fortunately it's not addictive.

The brain's/nervous systems are then poisoned, and have to shut down the entire ovarian functions, which are supposed to produce oestrogen, progesterone and androstenedione/

testosterone/DHEA to regulate the menstrual cycle and sexual/orgasmic functions. Now her body is flooded by the synthetic (or fake) progesterone. The effects can last for several years from just one shot.

The most effective treatment is to detoxify the liver and brain's nervous systems.

References

1. Whipple, Beverly (consultant), Schoen, Mark

(filmmaker). "Orgasmic expulsions of fluid in the sexually stimulated female." Film available from Focus International, Inc., 1776 Broadway, New York, N.Y.10019.

2. Darling, CA; Davidson, JK; Conway-Welch, C. (1990). "Female ejaculation: perceived origins, the Grafenberg spot/area, and sexual responsiveness.". *Arch Sex Behav* **19** (1): 29–47.

3. Addiego, F; Belzer, EG; Comolli, J; Moger, W; Perry, JD; Whipple, B. (1981). "Female ejaculation: a case study". *Journal of Sex Research* **17** (1): 13–21.

4. "The Orgasm Answer Guide" by Barry R. Komisaruk, Beverly Whipple, Sara Nasserzadeh, and Carlos Beyer-Flores. Baltimore: The Johns Hopkins University Press. 2010.

5. Whipple, Beverly, Eleanor Richards, Mitchell Tepper, and Barry R. Komisaruk. "Sexual Response in

Women with Complete Spinal Cord Injury." *Women with Physical Disabilities: Achieving and Maintaining Health and Well-Being*. Eds. Danuta M. Krotoski, Margaret A. Nosek, and Margaret A. Turk, eds Baltimore, MD: Paul H. Brookes Publishing Co., 1996. 69-80.

6. Heath D (1984). "An investigation into the origins of a copious vaginal discharge during intercourse: "Enough to wet the bed" – that "is not urine"". *J Sex Res.* **20** (2): 194–215.

7. Journal of the British Association for Sexual and Marital Therapy, Vol 12 No.4, November 1997

8. Mahler SV, Smith KS, Berridge KC (November 2007). "Endocannabinoid hedonic hotspot for sensory pleasure: anandamide in nucleus accumbens shell enhances 'liking' of a sweet reward". *Neuropsychopharmacology* **32** (11): 2267–78.

www.ingramcontent.com/pod-product-compliance
Lightning Source LLC
Chambersburg PA
CBHW070426290526
45791CB00005B/1852